Anti-Inflammatory Diet for Beginners

Essential Guide to Reducing Inflammation, Boosting Health, and Transforming Your Lifestyle with Wholesome Nutrition

Jimmy A. Jones

Table of Contents

Introduction

Understanding Inflammation

Importance of Anti-Inflammatory Diets

Chapter One: Basics of Inflammation

1.1 Inflammatory Processes in the Body

1.2 Chronic Inflammation and Health Risks

Chapter Two: Benefits of an Anti-Inflammatory Diet

2.1 Reducing Inflammation Naturally

2.2 Impact on Overall Health and Well-being

Chapter Three: Key Principles of Anti-Inflammatory Eating

3.1 Choosing the Right Foods

3.2 Foods to Avoid

Chapter Four: Foundation of an Anti-Inflammatory Diet

4.1 Whole Foods and Plant-Based Options

4.2 Importance of Omega-3 Fatty Acids

Chapter Five: Building Your Anti-Inflammatory Plate

5.1 Balanced Nutrition

5.2 Portion Control

Chapter Six: Anti-Inflammatory Recipes

6.1 Breakfast

6.2 Lunch

6.3 Dinner

6.4 Snacks and Desserts

Chapter Seven: Incorporating Anti-Inflammatory Herbs and Spices

7.1 Turmeric

7.2 Ginger

7.3 Garlic

Chapter Eight: Hydration and Anti-Inflammatory Drinks

8.1 Water and Herbal Teas

8.2 Detoxifying Beverages

Chapter Nine: Planning and Preparing Anti-Inflammatory Meals 9.1 Meal Planning Strategies

9.2 Grocery Shopping

Chapter Ten: Tips Addressing Common Challenges

10.1 Eating Out

10.2 Social Situations

Chapter Eleven: Maintaining an Anti-Inflammatory Lifestyle

11.1 Regular Physical Activity

11.2 Stress Management

Chapter Twelve: Tracking Progress
12.1 Monitoring Inflammatory Markers

12.2 Adjusting the Diet for Optimal Results

Chapter Thirteen: Frequently Asked Questions

13.1 Clarifying Misconceptions

14.2 Troubleshooting Common Issues

Conclusion

14.1 Recap of Key Points

14.2 Encouragement for Long-Term

Introduction
1.1 Understanding Inflammation
1.2 Importance of Anti-Inflammatory Diets

In the realm of health and wellness, the intricate dance between our bodies and inflammation takes center stage.

Understanding inflammation, denoted as 1.1, is paramount for anyone seeking to grasp the delicate balance within the human system. Inflammation, often misconceived as solely a negative force, is a fundamental biological response that the body initiates to protect itself from harmful stimuli. Whether triggered by injuries, infections, or chronic conditions, inflammation is the body's defense mechanism, albeit a double-edged sword.1.2 propels us into the crucial domain of anti-inflammatory diets, shedding light on the pivotal role nutrition plays in managing inflammation. The importance of anti-inflammatory diets transcends mere dietary choices; it is a holistic approach to nurturing the body and mitigating the impact of inflammatory responses. These diets prioritize foods rich in antioxidants, omega-3 fatty acids, and phytonutrients, which collectively contribute to reducing inflammation.The significance of comprehending inflammation and embracing anti-inflammatory diets lies not only in preventing diseases but also in optimizing overall well-being. As noted above, inflammation, when unregulated, can evolve into chronic conditions, becoming a driving force behind various health issues. The synergy between understanding inflammation and adopting anti-inflammatory diets empowers individuals to take proactive steps toward maintaining a balanced and resilient body.In this exploration, we delve into the intricacies of inflammation, unraveling its mysteries to appreciate its nuanced role in the body. Simultaneously, we navigate the landscape of anti-inflammatory diets, deciphering their impact on immune function and overall health. Together, these facets provide a comprehensive understanding of how lifestyle choices intertwine with the body's innate responses, offering a roadmap to a healthier, more harmonious existence.

Chapter One
Basics of Inflammation

1.1 Inflammatory Processes in the Body

1.2 Chronic Inflammation and Health Risks

Basics of Inflammation

Inflammation is a fundamental biological response that the body employs to protect itself from harmful stimuli, such as pathogens, damaged cells, or irritants. Chapter One delves into the intricacies of these inflammatory processes, shedding light on their significance in maintaining overall health.

1.1 Inflammatory Processes in the Body

The chapter initiates with a comprehensive exploration of the various inflammatory processes occurring within the human body. It elucidates how the immune system recognizes threats and mobilizes an intricate network of cells, proteins, and chemical signals to neutralize and eliminate potential dangers. This section provides a foundational understanding of the body's defense mechanisms and the orchestrated responses that occur at the cellular level. Readers will gain insights into acute inflammation, a rapid and self-limiting defense mechanism triggered by injuries or infections. The discussion extends to the involvement of white blood cells, such as neutrophils and macrophages, which play pivotal roles in identifying and eliminating foreign invaders. The chapter also explores the release of inflammatory mediators, including cytokines and chemokines, which orchestrate the immune response.

1.2 Chronic Inflammation and Health Risks

Moving beyond the acute phase, Chapter One scrutinizes the implications of chronic inflammation on overall health. Chronic inflammation, a persistent and prolonged response, is linked to a myriad of health risks. The chapter elucidates how sustained activation of the immune system can lead to tissue damage and contribute to the development of various diseases, including cardiovascular conditions, autoimmune disorders, and certain cancers. By delving into the intricacies of chronic inflammation, readers gain an understanding of the delicate balance required for a healthy immune response. The chapter emphasizes the importance of identifying and managing factors that contribute to chronic inflammation, such as lifestyle choices, diet, and environmental influences. As noted above, Chapter One provides a solid foundation for grasping the basics of inflammation, paving the way for subsequent chapters to explore specific aspects of this intricate biological process in greater detail.

Chapter Two
Benefits of an Anti-Inflammatory Diet

2.1   Reducing Inflammation Naturally

2.2 Impact on Overall Health and Well-being

Benefits of an Anti-Inflammatory Diet

In the pursuit of optimal health, understanding the benefits of an anti-inflammatory diet becomes paramount. This chapter delves into two key aspects: reducing inflammation naturally and the broader impact on overall health and well-being.

2.1 Reducing Inflammation Naturally

Inflammation, while a natural response to injury or infection, can become chronic and detrimental to health when it persists over time. An anti-inflammatory diet, rich in foods with proven anti-inflammatory properties, provides a natural and sustainable approach to mitigating this chronic inflammation. The inclusion of omega-3 fatty acids found in fatty fish, nuts, and seeds, coupled with antioxidants from fruits and vegetables, plays a pivotal role in quelling inflammation. Furthermore, herbs and spices like turmeric and ginger, known for their anti-inflammatory properties, can be incorporated into meals to enhance the diet's effectiveness. By adopting an anti-inflammatory diet, individuals may experience a reduction in inflammatory markers, contributing to improved joint health, decreased risk of chronic diseases, and enhanced overall bodily function. This natural approach not only addresses the symptoms but also tackles the root cause of inflammation, fostering long-term health benefits.2.2 Impact on Overall Health and Well-beingThe ripple effect of an anti-inflammatory diet extends far beyond inflammation control. Research suggests that such a dietary pattern positively influences various aspects of overall health and well-being. From bolstering the immune system to promoting cardiovascular health, the benefits are comprehensive. Individuals adhering to an anti-inflammatory diet often report increased energy levels, better mood, and improved cognitive function. Moreover, this dietary approach is associated with a reduced risk of chronic conditions such as heart disease, diabetes, and certain cancers. The anti-inflammatory diet's emphasis on whole, nutrient-dense foods aligns with a holistic approach to health, emphasizing the interconnectedness of bodily systems.In conclusion, Chapter Two explores the intrinsic benefits of adopting an anti-inflammatory diet. By naturally reducing inflammation and fostering overall health improvements, this dietary paradigm stands as a cornerstone for a vibrant and resilient life.

Chapter Three
Key Principles of Anti-Inflammatory Eating
3.1 Choosing the Right Foods

3.2 Foods to Avoid
Key Principles of Anti-Inflammatory Eating

In the pursuit of a healthier lifestyle, understanding the key principles of anti-inflammatory eating becomes paramount. This chapter delves into the fundamental aspects of selecting foods that promote a balanced and anti-inflammatory dict, while also highlighting those that should be avoided for optimal well-being.

3.1 Choosing the Right Foods

The foundation of anti-inflammatory eating lies in selecting foods known for their anti-inflammatory properties. Whole, nutrient-dense options such as fruits, vegetables, whole grains, and fatty fish are rich in antioxidants and essential nutrients. These elements play a crucial role in reducing inflammation and supporting overall health. Emphasizing a variety of colorful fruits and vegetables ensures a broad spectrum of beneficial compounds, each contributing to the body's natural defense against inflammation.Additionally, incorporating healthy fats, such as those found in olive oil, nuts, and avocados, provides anti-inflammatory benefits. These fats not only help regulate inflammation but also contribute to cardiovascular health. Including lean proteins and plant-based sources like legumes further adds to the diverse range of nutrients essential for maintaining an anti-inflammatory balance.

3.2 Foods to Avoid

Equally important to choosing the right foods is understanding which foods to limit or avoid. Processed foods high in refined sugars and trans fats are known to trigger inflammation. Reducing the consumption of these items not only curtails inflammation but also supports weight management and reduces the risk of chronic diseases. Furthermore, refined carbohydrates, commonly found in white bread and sugary snacks, should be minimized. These foods can cause spikes in blood sugar levels, leading to increased inflammation. Steering clear of excessive alcohol and processed meats also aligns with the principles of anti-inflammatory eating. In conclusion, Chapter Three serves as a comprehensive guide to navigating the intricacies of anti-inflammatory eating. By carefully selecting foods rich in nutrients and antioxidants while avoiding those known to promote inflammation, individuals can cultivate a diet that promotes overall well-being and resilience against inflammatory conditions.

Chapter Four
Foundation of an Anti-Inflammatory Diet

4.1 Whole Foods and Plant-Based Options

4.2 Importance of Omega-3 Fatty Acids

Foundation of an Anti-Inflammatory Diet

In the pursuit of optimal health, an anti-inflammatory diet stands out as a cornerstone strategy. Chapter Four delves into the foundational elements that shape this approach, emphasizing the significance of whole foods and plant-based options.

4.1 Whole Foods and Plant-Based Options

The essence of an anti-inflammatory diet lies in the conscious choice of whole, unprocessed foods. Fruits, vegetables, nuts, seeds, and legumes take center stage, offering a rich array of vitamins, minerals, and antioxidants. These nutrient-dense options contribute to the body's resilience against inflammation, fostering an internal environment that supports overall well-being. A key aspect highlighted in this chapter is the incorporation of plant-based alternatives. Plant-based diets have gained recognition for their potential to reduce inflammation, thanks to their abundance of phytochemicals and fiber. By focusing on these alternatives, individuals can not only mitigate inflammation but also promote cardiovascular health and maintain a healthy weight.

4.2 Importance of Omega-3 Fatty Acids

The spotlight then shifts to the critical role played by omega-3 fatty acids in maintaining an anti-inflammatory state. Found in fatty fish like salmon, walnuts, and flaxseeds, these essential fats contribute to the body's ability to regulate inflammation. The chapter elucidates on the various sources of omega-3s and their impact on inflammatory pathways, guiding readers towards incorporating these beneficial fats into their daily dietary practices. Understanding the importance of omega-3 fatty acids involves recognizing their anti-inflammatory and cardiovascular benefits. The chapter provides practical insights into integrating these nutrients into meals, empowering individuals to make informed choices for long-term health.In conclusion, Chapter Four serves as the bedrock for constructing an effective anti-inflammatory diet. By embracing whole foods, plant-based options, and recognizing the significance of omega-3 fatty acids, individuals are equipped

with the knowledge needed to foster a resilient
and inflammation-resistant lifestyle

Chapter Five
Building Your Anti-Inflammatory Plate
5.1 Balanced Nutrition

5.2 Portion Control

Building Your Anti-Inflammatory Plate

In the pursuit of optimal health and well-being, Chapter Five of our guide focuses on constructing an anti-inflammatory plate, emphasizing two critical aspects: Balanced Nutrition and Portion Control.

5.1 Balanced Nutrition

Achieving a well-rounded, anti-inflammatory diet begins with balanced nutrition. This entails incorporating a variety of nutrient-dense foods that promote overall health and combat inflammation. Emphasize colorful fruits and vegetables, which are rich in antioxidants, vitamins, and minerals essential for cellular repair. Include lean proteins, such as fish, poultry, and legumes, to provide a source of amino acids vital for muscle maintenance and immune function.Healthy fats play a crucial role in reducing inflammation. Incorporate sources like olive oil, avocados, and nuts, as they contain omega-3 fatty acids, known for their anti-inflammatory properties. Whole grains, like quinoa and brown rice, contribute fiber and complex carbohydrates, promoting digestive health and steady energy levels.

5.2 Portion Control

While consuming nutritious foods is pivotal, controlling portion sizes is equally important. Overeating, even with healthy foods, can lead to excess calorie intake and potential weight gain, which may exacerbate inflammation. Implementing portion control not only supports weight management but also allows the body to better utilize nutrients. Use visual cues, such as a palm-sized portion of protein, a fist-sized portion of carbohydrates, and a thumb-sized serving of healthy fats, to guide your meal composition. Listen to your body's hunger and fullness signals, eating mindfully to avoid overindulgence. Consider smaller, more frequent meals throughout the day to maintain stable blood sugar levels and prevent inflammatory responses triggered by large fluctuations. As noted above, achieving an anti-inflammatory plate requires a harmonious combination of diverse nutrients and mindful portion control. By embracing these principles, individuals can cultivate a sustainable and health-promoting eating pattern that not only fights inflammation but also supports overall wellness.

Chapter Six
Anti-Inflammatory Recipes

6.1 Breakfast

6.2 Lunch

6.3 Dinner

6.4 Snacks and Desserts

Chapter Six of our guide focuses on Anti-Inflammatory Recipes, providing a comprehensive approach to incorporating inflammation-fighting ingredients into every meal. This chapter is subdivided into four sections, each addressing a specific mealtime, to help you seamlessly integrate anti-inflammatory goodness into your daily diet.

6.1 Breakfast

Start your day with a burst of anti-inflammatory power. Explore recipes that feature ingredients like turmeric, ginger, and berries. Consider a turmeric-infused smoothie with fresh fruits or a chia seed pudding topped with antioxidant-rich berries. These breakfast options not only taste delightful but also contribute to reducing inflammation in the body.

6.2 Lunch

Lunchtime offers an opportunity to further enhance your anti-inflammatory journey. Incorporate leafy greens, lean proteins, and omega-3-rich foods into your midday meals. Try a colorful salad with spinach, salmon, and walnuts, or opt for a quinoa bowl loaded with veggies. These recipes not only satisfy your taste buds but also support overall well-being.

6.3 Dinner

As the day winds down, indulge in satisfying and anti-inflammatory dinners. Consider dishes with garlic, olive oil, and cruciferous vegetables. A roasted garlic and lemon chicken with a side of broccoli and quinoa provides a balanced and inflammation-fighting dinner option. These recipes promote a healthy lifestyle while ensuring a satisfying end to your day.

6.4 Snacks and Desserts

Craving a snack or a sweet treat? Choose options that align with the anti-inflammatory theme. Snack on nuts, seeds, and fresh fruit, or prepare a dessert with dark chocolate and berries. These alternatives not only curb your cravings but also contribute to reducing inflammation and promoting overall health. By embracing these Anti-Inflammatory Recipes for breakfast, lunch, dinner, and snacks/desserts, you are not only savoring delicious meals but also actively supporting your body's fight against inflammation. Make these recipes a part of your routine for a tasteful and health-conscious lifestyle.

Chapter Seven
Incorporating Anti-Inflammatory Herbs and Spices

7.1 Turmeric

7.2 Ginger

7.3 Garlic

Incorporating Anti-Inflammatory Herbs and Spices

In the pursuit of holistic well-being, Chapter Seven delves into the incorporation of anti-inflammatory herbs and spices, unveiling nature's potent remedies to combat inflammation. With a focus on three key players – turmeric, ginger, and garlic – this chapter provides invaluable insights into harnessing the therapeutic power of these culinary treasures.

7.1 Turmeric

Renowned for its vibrant hue and earthy flavor, turmeric stands out as a powerhouse in the anti-inflammatory realm. Its active compound, curcumin, boasts remarkable anti-inflammatory and antioxidant properties. This section explores various ways to integrate turmeric into your diet, from golden milk to curries, unlocking not only its distinct taste but also its potential to soothe inflammation and promote overall wellness.

7.2 Ginger

Moving on to ginger, a versatile spice celebrated for its zesty kick and medicinal properties, the chapter sheds light on its anti-inflammatory prowess. Known for containing gingerol, a bioactive compound, ginger can be a flavorful addition to dishes or enjoyed as a soothing tea. This section guides readers on creative ways to infuse ginger into their meals, emphasizing its role in supporting a healthy inflammatory response.

7.3 Garlic

Garlic, with its pungent aroma and robust flavor, emerges as another anti-inflammatory champion. Rich in allicin, a sulfur-containing compound, garlic possesses anti-inflammatory and immune-boosting attributes. The chapter explores diverse culinary applications of garlic, from sautéing in stir-fries to roasting in vegetable medleys, empowering readers to embrace this kitchen staple for both its taste and health benefits.As noted above, the content unfolds in a user-friendly manner, providing practical tips and delicious recipes to seamlessly incorporate turmeric, ginger, and garlic into everyday meals. By understanding and leveraging the anti-inflammatory properties of these herbs and spices, readers can embark on a flavorful journey towards improved well-being and vitality.

Chapter Eight
Hydration and Anti-Inflammatory Drinks
8.1 Water and Herbal Teas

8.2 Detoxifying Beverages

Hydration and Anti-Inflammatory Drinks explores the crucial role of beverages in maintaining overall health and well-being. This chapter delves into two key sections: 8.1 Water and Herbal Teas, and 8.2 Detoxifying Beverages.In section 8.1, the focus is on the fundamental element of hydration – water, and the benefits of herbal teas. Water, often overlooked, plays a pivotal role in bodily functions, from aiding digestion to regulating body temperature. The chapter emphasizes the significance of staying adequately hydrated for optimal health. Additionally, it explores the diverse world of herbal teas, known for their unique flavors and potential health benefits.

Whether it's chamomile for relaxation or peppermint for digestion, incorporating herbal teas into daily routines can enhance both hydration and overall wellness.Moving on to section 8.2, Detoxifying Beverages, the chapter discusses drinks specifically designed to promote detoxification and combat inflammation. Detoxifying beverages, such as infused water with citrus fruits or cucumber, are highlighted for their ability to flush out toxins and support the body's natural cleansing processes. The chapter provides insights into various recipes and ingredients that possess anti-inflammatory properties, contributing to a healthier lifestyle. Readers are guided through the science behind these drinks, understanding how they can help reduce inflammation and promote a balanced internal environment. The importance of choosing beverages rich in antioxidants and anti-inflammatory compounds is underscored, offering practical tips for integrating these drinks into daily routines.In conclusion, Chapter Eight serves as a comprehensive guide to the essential aspects of hydration and anti-inflammatory beverages. It equips readers with knowledge on the benefits of water, herbal teas, and detoxifying drinks, empowering them to make informed choices for a healthier and more balanced lifestyle.

Chapter Nine
Planning and Preparing Anti-Inflammatory Meals

9.1 Meal Planning Strategies

9.2 Grocery Shopping

Planning and Preparing Anti-Inflammatory

Meals dives into the crucial aspects of crafting meals that promote well-being and combat inflammation. This chapter unfolds with a comprehensive exploration of Meal Planning Strategies, a cornerstone in achieving dietary goals.

9.1 Meal Planning Strategies

Effective meal planning is a proactive approach to ensure a diet rich in anti-inflammatory elements. The chapter elucidates on the significance of incorporating a variety of colorful fruits, vegetables, whole grains, and lean proteins into daily meals. It emphasizes the balance between omega-3 and omega-6 fatty acids, encouraging the inclusion of sources like fatty fish, flaxseeds, and walnuts. The chapter further delves into the art of portion control, urging readers to be mindful of serving sizes to maintain a healthy caloric intake. It provides practical tips for structuring meals that are not only nutritionally sound but also enjoyable, fostering long-term adherence to an anti-inflammatory diet.

9.2 Grocery Shopping

Navigating the aisles with intentionality is pivotal in executing an anti-inflammatory meal plan. Section 9.2 sheds light on effective Grocery Shopping strategies, guiding readers on selecting fresh, whole foods while minimizing processed and inflammatory-inducing items. It underscores the importance of reading labels, identifying hidden sugars, and opting for organic produce when possible. The chapter champions the inclusion of spices like turmeric and ginger known for their anti-inflammatory properties. It educates readers on deciphering nutritional labels, making informed choices, and prioritizing nutrient-dense options during their shopping excursions. As noted above, the chapter integrates practical insights with scientific understanding, providing a holistic guide to planning and preparing meals that actively contribute to reducing inflammation. By focusing on Meal Planning Strategies and Grocery Shopping, readers are equipped with the knowledge and skills needed to transform their dietary habits positively .In essence, Chapter

Nine acts as a compass, steering individuals towards a path of wellness through thoughtful planning and mindful grocery choices.

Chapter Ten
Tips Addressing Common Challenges

10.1 Eating Out

10.2 Social Situations

Tips Addressing Common Challenges

In Chapter Ten of our comprehensive guide, we delve into practical strategies for navigating two common challenges: eating out and social situations. These scenarios often pose difficulties for individuals striving to maintain a particular lifestyle or adhere to specific dietary preferences. Our goal is to equip readers with actionable tips to overcome these hurdles gracefully.

10.1 Eating Out

Dining out can be a potential minefield for those aiming to make mindful food choices. However, armed with the right strategies, one can still enjoy restaurant meals without compromising their health goals. We recommend scanning menus in advance, looking for healthier options, and being clear about dietary restrictions when communicating with restaurant staff. Portion control is key, and opting for grilled or steamed dishes over fried alternatives can make a substantial difference. Additionally, cultivating the habit of savoring each bite mindfully allows for a more satisfying dining experience.

10.2 Social Situations

Social gatherings often revolve around food and drinks, making them challenging for individuals with specific dietary preferences. This section provides insights on gracefully navigating such situations. One valuable tip is to plan ahead by eating a nutritious snack before attending an event, reducing the temptation to indulge in less healthy options. Communication is crucial; informing hosts or friends about dietary restrictions can lead to accommodations and a more enjoyable experience for everyone. For those facing peer pressure, learning to assertively express one's choices without making others uncomfortable is a valuable skill. Additionally, bringing a dish to share ensures there's at least one option aligned with personal dietary goals. As noted above, these practical tips aim to empower individuals in addressing common challenges related to eating out and social situations. By implementing these strategies, readers can confidently navigate various scenarios, maintaining control over their choices and well-being.

Chapter Eleven
Maintaining an Anti-Inflammatory Lifestyle

11.1 Regular Physical Activity

11.2 Stress Management

Maintaining an Anti-Inflammatory Lifestyle

In the pursuit of overall well-being, Chapter Eleven delves into the critical aspects of maintaining an anti-inflammatory lifestyle, focusing on two key elements: Regular Physical Activity and Stress Management.

11.1 Regular Physical Activity

Regular physical activity is a cornerstone of an anti-inflammatory lifestyle. Engaging in exercise not only promotes cardiovascular health and weight management but also plays a pivotal role in reducing inflammation within the body. Physical activity triggers the release of endorphins, known as "feel-good" hormones, which contribute to stress reduction and overall mental well-being. From brisk walks to intense workouts, incorporating regular exercise into daily routines is paramount for combating chronic inflammation.Research consistently highlights the positive impact of exercise on inflammatory markers. It not only helps regulate the immune system but also enhances insulin sensitivity, reducing the risk of chronic diseases associated with inflammation. Whether through aerobic activities, strength training, or flexibility exercises, the key is consistency. Integrating physical activity into one's lifestyle becomes a proactive approach to mitigating inflammation and fostering a healthier body.

11.2 Stress Management

Stress, a pervasive element of modern life, is a significant contributor to chronic inflammation. Chapter Eleven underscores the importance of effective stress management strategies in maintaining an anti-inflammatory lifestyle. Chronic stress triggers the release of cortisol, a hormone associated with inflammation. Thus, adopting stress-reducing techniques is crucial for long-term health. Various approaches, such as mindfulness meditation, deep breathing exercises, and yoga, are explored within this chapter. These practices not only calm the mind but also have tangible physiological effects, lowering inflammatory markers. By cultivating a mindset that embraces stress management as an integral part of overall health, individuals can create a protective shield against the detrimental effects of chronic inflammation. In conclusion, Chapter Eleven guides readers through the pivotal components of an anti-inflammatory lifestyle. Regular physical activity and effective stress management serve as powerful tools in the pursuit of optimal health, offering not only immediate benefits but also long-term resilience against inflammation-related disorders.

Chapter Twelve
Tracking Progress

12.1 Monitoring Inflammatory Markers

12.2 Adjusting the Diet for Optimal Results

Tracking Progress

In the journey towards optimal health, Chapter Twelve serves as a pivotal guide, focusing on "Tracking Progress." This chapter delves into two key aspects that play a crucial role in gauging and enhancing one's well-being: monitoring inflammatory markers and adjusting the diet for optimal results.

12.1 Monitoring Inflammatory Markers

Understanding and managing inflammation is vital for overall health. Section 12.1 introduces the concept of monitoring inflammatory markers, shedding light on their significance in assessing the body's response to various factors. By closely observing markers such as C-reactive protein (CRP) and interleukin-6, individuals gain insights into the inflammatory state within their bodies. Regular tracking of inflammatory markers allows for early detection of potential health issues and aids in creating targeted interventions. The chapter emphasizes the importance of consulting healthcare professionals to interpret these markers accurately. Whether it's adopting an anti-inflammatory diet or incorporating lifestyle changes, the goal is to keep inflammation at bay, promoting long-term well-being.

12.2 Adjusting the Diet for Optimal Results

Section 12.2 focuses on the intricate relationship between diet and health outcomes. It underscores the need for a personalized approach, recognizing that each individual's nutritional requirements vary. The chapter explores methods of fine-tuning diets based on specific health goals, metabolic responses, and dietary preferences.Adjusting the diet for optimal results involves not only choosing nutrient-dense foods but also understanding how certain foods may contribute to or mitigate inflammation. The chapter encourages readers to experiment with dietary changes, closely monitoring how these adjustments influence overall health and well-being.In conclusion, Chapter Twelve provides a comprehensive roadmap for individuals seeking to optimize their health journey. By monitoring inflammatory markers and adjusting the diet for optimal results, readers are equipped with valuable tools to track and enhance their progress towards a healthier, more vibrant life.

Chapter Thirteen
Frequently Asked Questions

13.1 Clarifying Misconceptions

14.2 Troubleshooting Common Issues
Frequently Asked Questions

In Chapter Thirteen, we delve into addressing common queries and concerns, aiming to provide clarity and solutions for a smoother user experience.

13.1 Clarifying Misconceptions

This section focuses on dispelling common misunderstandings that users may encounter. By addressing misconceptions head-on, we aim to enhance user understanding and reduce any potential frustration. Whether it's clarifying the purpose of specific features or debunking myths associated with the product, this chapter serves as a comprehensive guide to set the record straight.Through concise explanations and straightforward language, users will find answers to questions they might not have realized they had. From unraveling technical jargon to offering insights into product functionalities, this section serves as a reliable resource for users seeking accurate information.

13.2 Troubleshooting Common Issues

In the troubleshooting segment of Chapter Thirteen, we tackle prevalent problems that users may face. By providing step-by-step solutions and insights into resolving issues, we empower users to navigate challenges effectively. From software glitches to connectivity hiccups, this section acts as a troubleshooter's guide, equipping users with the knowledge to overcome obstacles. Each problem addressed in this chapter is accompanied by detailed instructions, ensuring that users can follow along easily. Troubleshooting tips are presented in a logical sequence, facilitating a systematic approach to problem-solving. By emphasizing user-friendly solutions, this chapter reinforces the idea that technical hurdles can be overcome with the right guidance. Chapter Thirteen is not just a compendium of information but a practical toolkit for users, promoting a positive and informed interaction with the product. Whether users seek to understand the intricacies of the system or resolve pesky issues hindering their experience, this chapter stands as a valuable resource in enhancing user satisfaction and overall product engagement.

Conclusion

In conclusion, a recap of key points serves as a vital tool for reinforcing the main ideas discussed throughout the content. By revisiting these essential concepts, readers gain a comprehensive understanding of the subject matter. In this context, it allows us to reflect on the journey undertaken in the preceding sections.Section 14.1, "Recap of Key Points," plays a pivotal role in cementing the foundation of knowledge. As we revisit the core elements, we not only reinforce our understanding but also provide a concise summary for those who may have missed certain details. This recap serves as a mental checklist, ensuring that the audience leaves with a clear and cohesive grasp of the information presented.Furthermore, Section 14.2, "Encouragement for Long-Term," emphasizes the importance of sustaining the momentum gained from the insights shared. It is not merely about understanding the key points momentarily but embracing them as part of a long-term commitment. Encouragement is the driving force that propels individuals to apply the knowledge gained consistently over time.Encouraging long-term engagement with the subject matter fosters a sense of dedication and perseverance. Whether it be implementing new practices, adopting a different mindset, or honing specific skills, the encouragement for long-term commitment ensures that the benefits extend beyond the immediate context. This section serves as a motivational catalyst, inspiring individuals to embark on a continuous journey of growth and improvement.In conclusion, the combination of recapping key points and offering encouragement for the long term creates a dynamic conclusion that reinforces understanding while motivating sustained engagement. As we bring this content to a close, let us carry forward the distilled wisdom and inspiration, applying it not just in the present moment but as a guiding force in the journey ahead.